Alia Jebri
Hager Sabta

Assessment of knowledge of cardiac arrest management

Alia Jebri
Hager Sabta

Assessment of knowledge of cardiac arrest management

Contribution of simulation-based learning

ScienciaScripts

Imprint
Any brand names and product names mentioned in this book are subject to trademark, brand or patent protection and are trademarks or registered trademarks of their respective holders. The use of brand names, product names, common names, trade names, product descriptions etc. even without a particular marking in this work is in no way to be construed to mean that such names may be regarded as unrestricted in respect of trademark and brand protection legislation and could thus be used by anyone.

Cover image: www.ingimage.com

This book is a translation from the original published under ISBN 978-620-3-42627-4.

Publisher:
Sciencia Scripts
is a trademark of
Dodo Books Indian Ocean Ltd., member of the OmniScriptum S.R.L Publishing group
str. A.Russo 15, of. 61, Chisinau-2068, Republic of Moldova Europe
Printed at: see last page
ISBN: 978-620-4-13134-4

Table of Contents

List of Abbreviations

TSA: Senior Anaesthesia Technician

MAR : Physician in Anaesthesia Intensive Care

TSAF : Trained Superior Technician in Anesthesia

RTA: Cardiopulmonary arrest

AC: Cardiac arrest

CPR: Cardiopulmonary Resuscitation

VF: Ventricular Fibrillation

VT: Ventricular **Tachycardia**

AED: Automated External Defibrillator

ECG: Electrocardiogram

EEC: External Electric Shock

IVD: Intravenous Direct

AEssP: Pulseless Electrical Activity

SpO2: Pulse Oxygen Saturation

FiO2: Fraction of inspired **oxygen**

RF: Respiratory Rate

Vt : Tidal volume

IO: Intra Bone

ACBO : Cardiac arrest in the operating room

PetCO2: Carbon dioxide tele-expiratory pressure

EG : Gas Embolism

CO2: Carbon dioxide

N2O: nitrous oxide

Introduction

Cardiac arrest, also known as sudden adult death or cardiopulmonary arrest, is an abrupt cessation of heart muscle contractions and breathing by the patient, resulting in an interruption of perfusion to the body's vital organs.

Cardiac arrest (CA) remains a major public health problem in industrialized countries, affecting more than 420,000 patients annually in the USA. In France, it is estimated that between 30,000 and 50,000 cardiac arrests occur each year [1].

For health professionals, recognition of cardiac arrest is based on the absence of signs of circulation (absence of signs of life and absence of central carotid or femoral pulses), the management of cardiac arrest in hospital must first follow the principles of the algorithms emanating from international and national recommendations.

Failure to recover electrical activity of the heart after stroke is often due to lack of prompt management of the victim, mainly because of delayed diagnosis.

Survival then depends on the speed of resuscitation. Cardiac arrest does not necessarily mean death if the right precautions were taken at the right time.

Simulation training is currently used in the health sector, allowing participants to be put in real-life conditions.

The importance of training all health care personnel in first aid is necessary and simulation plays a fundamental role in this training.

. Purpose of this research :

. To evaluate the knowledge of anesthesia and resuscitation technicians and physicians regarding the management of a cardiopulmonary arrest occurring in the operating room

. To promote the interest of training by simulation concerning cardiorespiratory arrest in order to refresh the knowledge and develop the skills of the interveners.

Materials and methods

Type and location of the study:

This is a prospective, analytical and evaluative study in the form of an anonymous, multi-centre questionnaire. We distributed 100 questionnaires to anaesthesia staff (doctors and technicians) in the following hospitals

The Main Military Hospital of Instruction of Tunis

. Charles Nicolle Hospital

. La Rabta Hospital

. Private clinics (El Yosr (Gafsa), Pasteur, Amen La Marsa, Montplaisir)

Fifty questionnaires distributed to anesthetists and physicians trained in simulation-based RTA management and 50 questionnaires for those not trained in simulation.

Study period:

Our study lasted 2 months (from March 1st to April 30th)

Inclusion criteria:

- Senior Anaesthesia Technician (SAT) working in the operating theatre

- Anaesthesiologist (MAR).

Study protocol:

We prepared and distributed a questionnaire (Appendix 4) with the following parts:

4.1 Characteristics of the participants:

. Hospital

. Sex

. Function

. Seniority in grade

4.2 The questions asked explored the following themes:

. Participation in a specific simulation training on cardiac arrest

. Early detection of cardiac arrest

. The precise approach to care

. Etiologies and reversible causes of RTA

. Appropriate post-arrest management

Ethical consideration:

The consent of the head of department and the anaesthetists in each department

* Anonymity of the participants

Statistical analysis:

The data was entered using Microsoft Excel and analyzed using SPSS version 23.

The results were expressed as numbers and percentages.

A chi-square test was used for the comparative study and the significance level was set at 0.05.

RESULTS

Results

Descriptive study :

1. *Distribution by place of work :*

Most of the respondents (33%) were practicing at the El Yosr clinic in Gafsa (Figure 1).

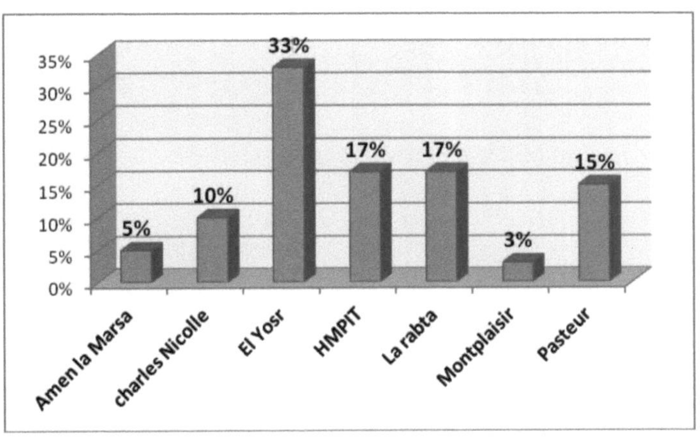

Figure 1: Distribution by place of work

Gender distribution :

The gender distribution of the study population shows a predominance of 68% women.

Study population:

In our study population, simulation training interested 49.4% of ASDs, 57.1% of anesthesia

residents and 50% of senior anesthesia residents (Figure 2).

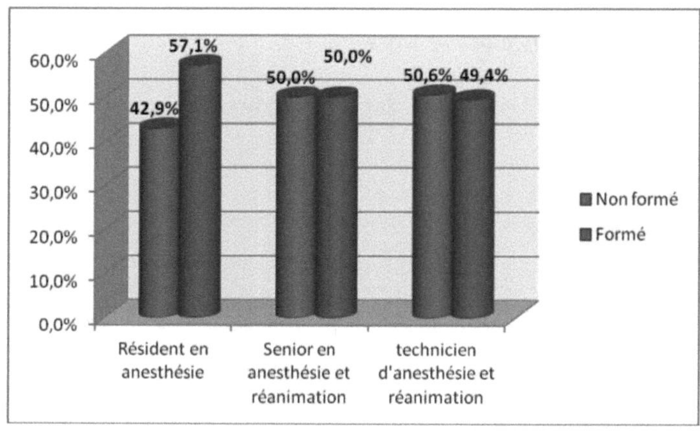

Figure 2: Distribution by status

Distribution by seniority :

Thirty-nine (39%) of the staff had a seniority of less than 5 years, while 40% had a seniority of more than 10 years (Figure 3).

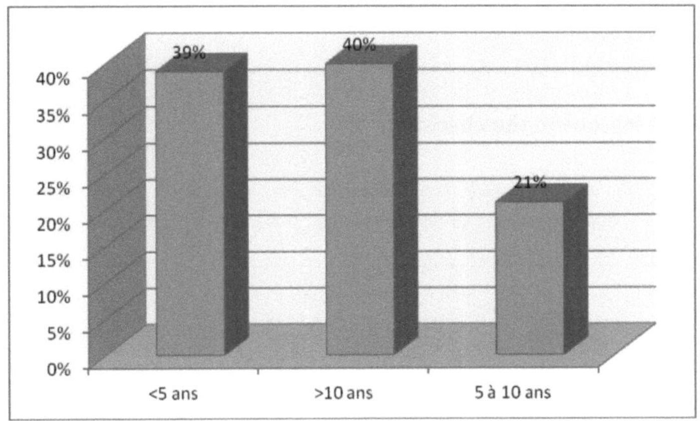

Figure 3: Distribution by seniority

Analytical study:

1.   Participation in a training session on ACBO:

Half of the respondents had had specific training in RTA.

Special feature in the checklist:

Of those trained in simulation, 88% stated that there were specifics in the checklist while 78% in the untrained group were aware of these specifics (p =0.14). (Figure 4)

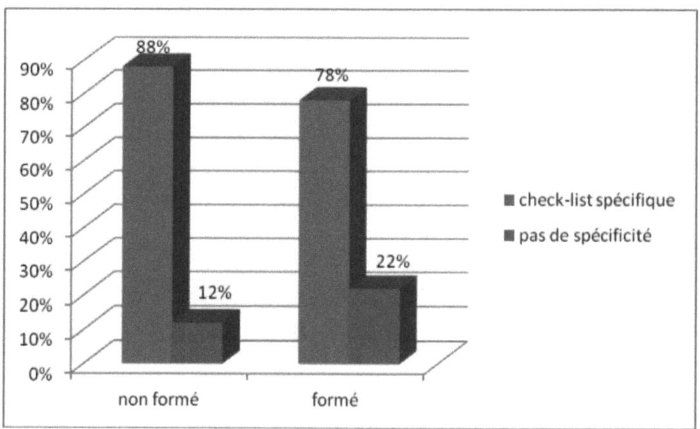

Figure 4: Special feature in the checklist

2.1 Checklist items :

Among the trained, 74% answered correctly to the checklist items namely defibrillator and emergency drugs (42%) while only 52% cited the defibrillator and 36% cited emergency drugs among the untrained (Table 1).

	Untrained	Formed	P
Defibrillator on	52%	74%	
Emergency drugs	36%	42%	
Incorrect answer	8%	10%	0,15
No response	12%	2%	

Table 1: Features of the checklist

Staff with a history of RTA :

The following table shows that 88% of the trained participants and 78% of the untrained participants have already managed a victim of cardiac arrest (p=0.27) (Table 2).

	Untrained	Formed	P
No	22%	12%	
Yes	78%	88%	0,27

Table 2: Participants who have had an RTA

The first warning sign of cardiac arrest in the operating room:

Of the trained participants, 10% answered incorrectly while 24% of the untrained participants did not give the correct answer.

The first warning sign of intraoperative cardiac arrest was hypocapnia for 46% of the trained patients versus 22% of the untrained patients.
Other responses were detection of asystole, bradycardia, desaturation and unstoppable blood pressure (Table 3)

	Not trained	Formed	P
No response	10%	6%	
Incorrect answer	24%	10%	
Hypocapnia	22%	46%	
Asystole	26%	22%	0,09
Bradycardia	24%	24%	
Desaturation	16%	18%	
Unbeatable blood pressure	4%	10%	

Table 3: Detection of RTA intraoperatively

Etiologies of cardiac arrest at induction :

Among the trained, 12% mentioned vagal discomfort as the main etiology of cardiac arrest at induction and 64% mentioned shock as the cause while among the untrained shock was the main cause of cardiac arrest at induction (52%) followed

by vagal discomfort (2%), this difference was not statistically significant. (Table 4)

	Untrained	Formed	P
State of shock	52%	64%	
Vagal discomfort	2%	12%	
Poisoning	0%	10%	0,23
Incorrect answer	22%	14%	
No response	24%	6%	

Table 4: Causes of cardiac arrest at induction

What to do in the event of cardiac arrest :

Regardless of whether participants were trained or not, only 60% responded
that they would initiate CPR in the face of a CPR event, and the rate of
participants who discontinued anesthesia was almost nil.
Only 8% of the trained and 16% of the untrained call for help in the event of an
RTA in the operating room, although the difference between the two groups is
not significant (p=0.32) (Figure 5).

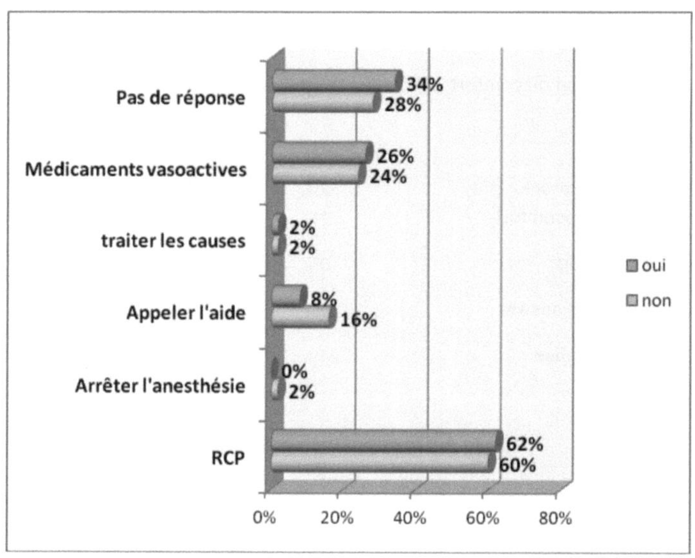

Figure 5: What to do in the event of cardiac arrest

Number of chest compressions during CPR :

Of the respondents who had received simulation training, 82% responded that the number of chest compressions was 30 versus 42% of the untrained group. This difference was statistically significant (p=0.01).

The compression/ventilation ratio:

Ninety (90%) of the trained participants practiced a 30:2 ratio between compressions and ventilations while only 64% of the other group applied this ratio, this difference was statistically significant (p=0.01).

Ventilation of the RTA patient :

There was no significant difference in the ventilation of the cardiac arrest patient between the trained and untrained groups. (Table 5)

	Untrained	Formed	P
No response	8%	6%	
Vt: 10-12 ml/kg, Inspiratory rate: 40/min, Insp time: 3 sec	22%	24%	
Vt: 4-5ml/k9, Inspiratory rate: 6/mn, Time: 1 sec	16%	14%	0,96
Vt: 6-7 ml/kg, Inspiratory rate: 10/min, Insp time: 2 sec	54%	56%	

Table 5: Ventilation of a CA patient

The proper depth of chest compressions for an adult to receive effective CPR:

The majority of the trained participants (78%) answered the question correctly by choosing a depth of 5-6 cm while 60% of the untrained participants answered correctly. The difference between the two groups was statistically significant (p=0.03). (Table 6)

	Untrained	Formed	P
10 to 15 cm	0%	4%	
5 to 6 cm	60%	78%	
6 to 10 cm	34%	18%	
No response	6%	0%	0,03

Table 6: Proper depth of chest compressions

The frequency of CPR compressions:

In the trained group, 68% gave a correct response of 100 to 120/min versus 28% in the untrained group. (Table 7)

	Untrained	Formed	P
100 to 120 /min	28%	68%	
50 to 60/ min	44%	24%	
75 to 80 /min	20%	6%	0,1
No response	8%	2%	

Table 7: Frequency of chest compressions

CPR may be discontinued if hypothermia occurs:

The majority of respondents, 88% in the simulation training group and 82% in the untrained group, responded that resuscitation should not be interrupted in case of hypothermia (p=0.32). (Table 8)

	1-Training		p
	Untrained	Formed	
No	82%	88%	
Yes	18%	10%	
No response	0%	2%	0,32

Table 8: Discontinue CPR if hypothermia

The drug of choice for cardiac arrest:

In our study, 100% of the trained participants used adrenaline as the drug of choice in cardiac arrest and 98% of the untrained group chose this response (p=0.5).

13.1   The right dose:

Ninety (90%) of the trained staff and 72% of the untrained responded that the dose

of epinephrine to be administered was 1 mg (p=0.04) (Table 9).

	Untrained	Formed	P
1 mg	72%	90%	
No response	22%	10%	0,04
incorrect response	6%	0%	

Table 9: Adequate Dose of Epinephrine

13.2   Drug administration cycle:

Sixty (60%) of the well-trained respondents answered that epinephrine should be administered every 2 cycles cf CPR versus 40% of the untrained respondents (p=0.04) (Table 10).

	Untrained	Formed	P
2 cycles	30%	60%	
3 cycles	18%	8%	
4 cycles	40%	32%	0,04
No response	12%	0%	

Table 10: Drug Administration Cycle

Administration of an antiarrhythmic drug:

Among the respondents trained by simulation, 82% answered that the administration of an antiarrhythmic should be done after the 3rd or 4th ERC versus 62% in the untrained group, this difference was not statistically significant (Table 11).

	Untrained	Formed	P
Before the 3rd or 4th external electric shock	24%	10%	
After the 3rd or 4th external electric shock	62%	82%	0,85
No response	14%	6%	

Table 11: Administration of an antiarrhythmic drug

Type of defibrillator:

In the fields studied in our survey, 68% use an automated external defibrillator and

14% use a semi-automatic defibrillator.

Definition of a shockable rhythm:

The shockable rhythms were ventricular fibrillation for 44% of the trained versus

66% in the untrained group and ventricular tachycardia for 70% of the trained

versus 48% in the untrained group (p=0.07) (Table 12).

	Untrained	Formed	P
Ventricular fibrillation	66%	44%	
Ventricular tachycardia	48%	70%	
Incorrect answer	2%	0%	0,07
No response	32%	8%	

Table 12: Shockable rhythms

First gesture after delivering the shock:

In the trained group, 66% resumed CPR immediately after an ERC while only 38% in the untrained group resumed CPR after the ERC, this difference was not statistically significant (Table 13).

	Training		P
	Untrained	Formed	
No response	36%	10%	
Incorrect answer	26%	24%	0 ,5
Resume CPR	38%	66%	

Table 13: First action after delivering the shock

Reversible causes of cardiac arrest:

A majority ranging from 62% to 78% of trained respondents correctly cited the reversible causes of cardiac arrest, this percentage ranged from 24% to 48% for untrained respondents (p=0.08) (Figure 6).

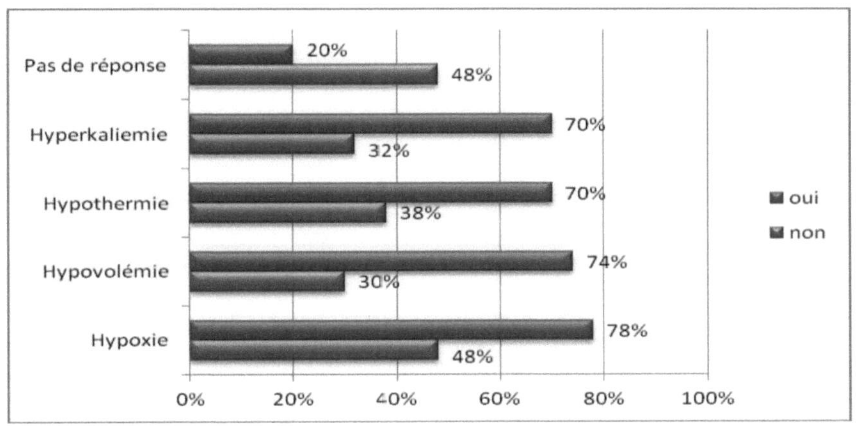

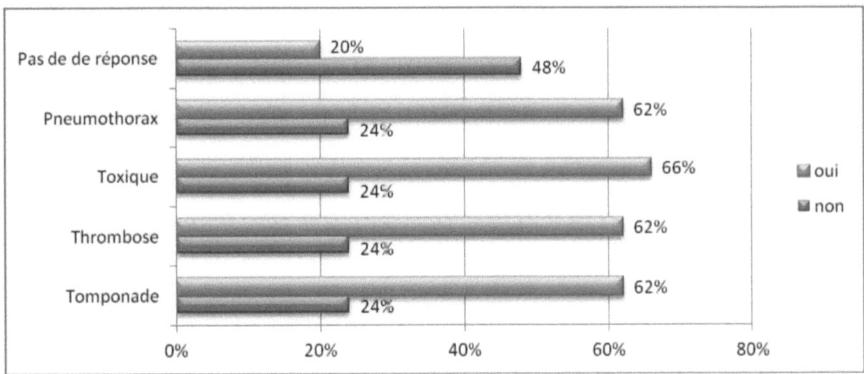

Figure 6: Reversible causes of CA

Causes of cardiac arrest during laparoscopy:

A rate of 70% of the trained population cited gas embolism as a cause of CA

during laparoscopy versus 54% for the untrained population.   (Figure 7)

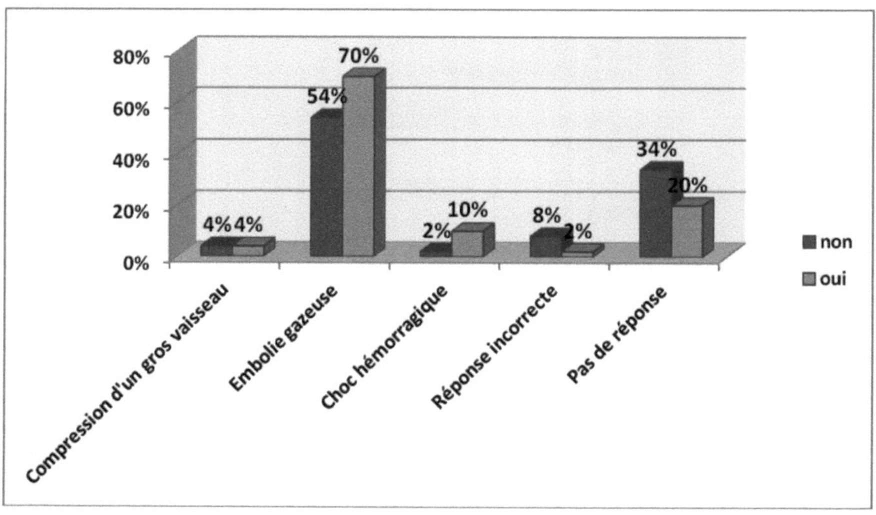

Figure 7: Causes of CA during laparoscopy

Specific care in the post-cardiac arrest period:

Thirty (30%) of the surveyed participants who had simulation training cited hemodynamic stability as the primary resuscitative measure after CA recovery followed by neuroprotection (14%) and maintenance of homeostasis (8%). The rate of untrained respondents who maintained hemodynamic stability and provided neuroprotection was lower (Table 13).

	Untrained	Formed	P
Stabilize hemodynamic status	10%	30%	
Maintaining homeostasis	24%	8%	
Neuroprotection	2%	14%	0,35
Incorrect answer	8%	4%	
No response	32%	22%	

DISCUSSION

Discussion:

ACBO is a serious complication of anesthesia that increases morbidity and mortality. Knowledge of the warning signs and the appropriate course of action is necessary for health professionals working in the operating room, especially ASD and MAR.

The occurrence of CA while the patient is intubated, artificially ventilated and monitored changes the course of action.

Intraoperative monitoring, which is mandatory for all patients in the operating room, should allow for immediate diagnosis or even anticipation or prevention of CA. In all cases, there should be no delay before the start of cardiopulmonary resuscitation (CPR).

Thus, the lack of delay makes the prognosis more favorable than for out-of-hospital CA.

1.   The checklist and its specificities :

In 2008, the World Health Organization (WHO) created a tool aimed at reducing deaths in surgical departments: the checklist. The implementation of a checklist has been associated with a reduction in mortality and complication rates in patients aged 16 years or older who underwent non-cardiac surgery [2].

Among the items in the CA checklist, the emergency cart is an important element. It must contain all the equipment necessary for the proper management of a life-threatening emergency, such as the drugs and fluids necessary for resuscitation. These trolleys are exclusively dedicated to the management of life-threatening emergencies, and must be accessible 24 hours a day, and their location must be indicated and known to everyone [3].

The second thing to check is the working defibrillator. It must always be available and accessible in case of an AC.

In 2016, the French Society of Anesthesia and Resuscitation (SFAR) launched a Cognitive Aids project, this project aimed to improve the medical and paramedical performance of the team in the management of the patient in critical and rare events, including cognitive aid sheets for the management of cardiac arrest in asystole and shockable rhythm (Appendix 2 , 3). These cognitive aids are made available to the nursing staff in the operating room. For ASD and MAR, the proper use of these cognitive aids requires simulation training [4].

The results of our study concerning the presence of specificity in the checklist, the majority of the respondents of both trained and untrained populations (88% and 78%) confirmed the presence of specificity in the checklist.

The untrained respondents did not manage to mention all the features of the checklist, only 52% mentioned the defibrillator and 36% mentioned the emergency drugs.

Although a significant proportion of the staff interviewed had more than 10 years' experience in the field and had had cardiac arrest training, simulation training facilitates learning and anchors knowledge.

2.   ACBO diagnosis:

Patient monitoring plays a crucial role in the positive diagnosis. The use of the electrocardiographic trace on the scope allows the positive diagnosis of RTA by highlighting its initial rhythm.

The monitoring of exhaled carbon dioxide with measurement of the tele-expiratory pressure in CO_2 is a major tool in the diagnosis of circulatory inefficiency. Indeed, the expired CO_2 pressure appears to be a reflection of the cardiac output due to a decrease in pulmonary perfusion and therefore an increase in the alveolar dead space, at constant ventilation and cellular metabolism. Thus, a sudden drop in PETCO2 should suggest a circulatory change, which sometimes precedes RTA, when PETCO2 will tend towards 0 mm Hg. Other causes of zero PETCO2 such as oesophageal intubation, circuit disconnection or bronchospasm should be ruled out [5].

Therefore, during any anaesthesia (general or locoregional) the patient should be scoped with an electrocardiographic monitor, a pulse oximeter, a non-invasive blood pressure device and a capnograph.

3.   Chest compressions:

Chest compressions generate sufficient blood flow to achieve cardiac and cerebral perfusion. Compressions performed with arms outstretched and hands positioned over the lower half of the patient's sternum [6].

The recommended technique for chest compressions calls for 30 compressions at a rate of 100-120/min to a depth of at least 5-6 cm in adults but not more than 6 cm [6].

Thus, survival is correlated with the number of adequate chest compressions performed at the correct frequency.

When artificial ventilation is combined with external cardiac massage, the ratio of chest compressions to artificial ventilation is 30:2 in adults. Because external cardiac massage is tiring, it is associated with a decrease in the quality of CPR over time, which is why it is recommended that a relay be performed between CPR participants, with the shortest possible interruption in cardiac massage.

Any interruption of chest compressions results in a decrease in survival [7].

In our study, among the respondents who had simulation training, the rate of participants knowing these specifics of chest compression, i.e., number of compressions, frequency, depth, and compression-ventilation ratio was significantly greater than that of the untrained population.

Simulation training is thus superior to theoretical knowledge alone. As chest compressions are a priority in resuscitation, it is important to practice to master the technique of compressions, so simulation allows to acquire these skills and improve practices.

4.   Ventilation:

4.1   Intubated/ventilated patient:

The correct endotracheal position of the tube should be confirmed first by different methods (appearance and number of cycles of capnography, auscultation of the pulmonary flaps), including in particular the capnography curve. The recommendations insist on the interest of continuous quantitative capnography in intubated patients throughout the peri-AC period, as this technique allows both to confirm the correct endotracheal positioning of the intubation tube, and to monitor the quality of CPR [8].

After tracheal intubation, mechanical ventilation is performed with a ventilator in controlled assisted ventilation mode, with a tidal volume of 6 to 7 ml/kg, a respiratory rate of 10 cycles/min, and a FiO2 of 100% during CPR.

In our study, whether or not the staff were trained by simulation, a low rate (54% for the untrained and 56% for the trained) chose the appropriate parameters for patient ventilation.

Indeed, even in simulation training, ventilation settings are not always addressed in a practical way.

4.2   Patient not yet intubated/ventilated:

The upper airway (UAV) must be opened by tilting the head back and raising the chin, with control of the permeability of the UAV to prevent hypoxic lesions, and is performed in the first instance using a manual insufflator and a mask, connected to an oxygen source.

Regardless of the ventilation technique used, the duration of insufflation is one second. The volume insufflated must be sufficient to lift the chest.

5.   Pharmacological treatment:

5.1 Adrenalin Square:

Epinephrine is the key drug in the management of cardiac arrest, primarily because of its vasoconstrictive alpha-adrenergic effect to improve coronary and cerebral perfusion during CPR.

High doses of epinephrine, while improving survival, are associated with a high rate of complications post-Acutephalus, which is why they are no longer recommended.

The recommended dosage of epinephrine during medical CPR remains 1 mg IV or IO, every 4 minutes, which corresponds to 2 cycles of CPR [9].

All trained and untrained respondents (100% and 98%) confirmed that the drug of choice during CA was Adrenaline.

But only 60% of trained staff and 30% of untrained staff administer Adrenalin every 2 cycles.

During simulation training, the acquisition of the CPR algorithm and the timing of epinephrine administration is easier to remember.

5.2 Place of antiarrhythmics:
The molecule currently recommended as first-line therapy for VF or VT refractory to electric

shocks is Amiodarone, administered as a bolus of 300 mg IV or IO after the 3rd electric shock, if necessary renewed as a 2nd bolus of 150 mg IV or IO after the 5th shock [10].

Lidocaine is no longer recommended as a first-line treatment for VF or VT, it is an alternative to Amiodarone when the latter is not available, and in this case should be administered at a dosage of 1 to 1.5 mg/kg IV or IO.

On the other hand, Lidocaine should not be used if Amiodarone has been previously injected without success [10].

In our study, 82% of the trained respondents answered that the administration of an antiarrhythmic should be done after the 3rd or 4th external shock, a percentage of 62% of the other untrained respondents gave the same answer showing the role of simulation training to update knowledge and adapt to new recommendations.

6.   Defibrillation:

Defibrillation is used in the event of ventricular fibrillation or pulseless ventricular tachycardia to help restore spontaneous circulation.

6.1   Shockable rhythms:

The shockable rhythms are Ventricular Tachycardia (VT) and Ventricular Fibrillation (VF).

If asystole is present, ERCs cannot be issued (Appendix 2)

VFs are defined by anarchic, desynchronized and inefficient contractions of the myocardial muscle [7] (Figure 8).

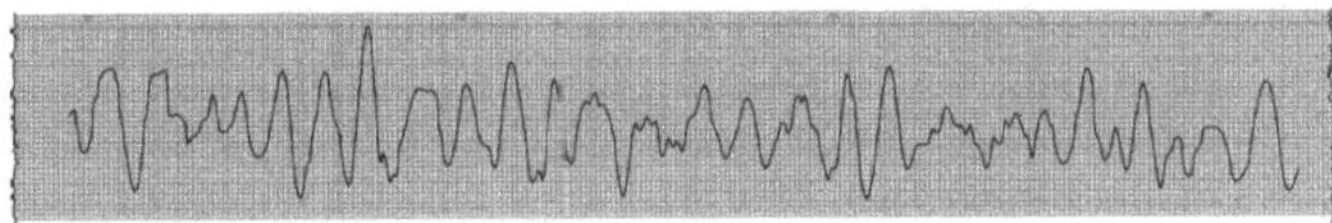

Figure 8: Ventricular Fibrillation

VTs are defined by a regular wide QRS tachycardia that spontaneously progresses to secondary VFs [7] (Figure 9).

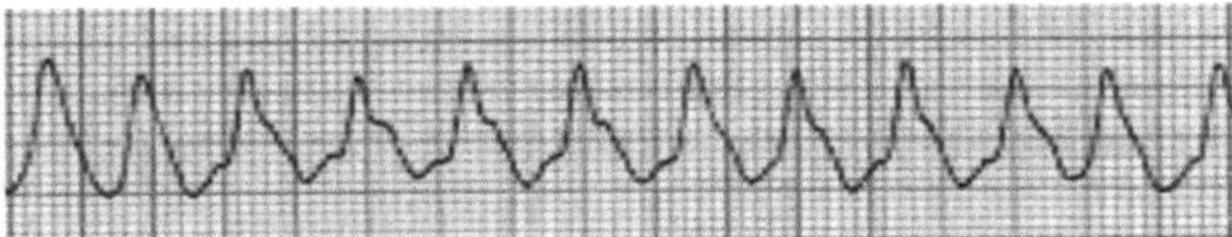

Figure 9: Ventricular Tachycardia

The survival and functional prognosis of BACO is significantly better when it occurs in VT or VF, 37% of patients survive after BACO in VF, a comparable figure for VT, whereas only 11% of patients found in asystole leave the hospital alive. There is no difference between VT and VF [7].

In our study, 70% of the trained anaesthetists answered that the shockable rhythms were VT and 44% of them also mentioned VF, while 34% of the untrained technicians gave an incorrect answer or did not answer.

The ACBO is a rare but serious complication, an erroneous conduct in front of a shockable rhythm worsens the prognosis, introducing the simulation as a training method allows all the health professionals in the operating room to intervene in time during an AC with shockable rhythm, it will allow to know the various tracings of TV and VF for which one carries out a CEE but also to learn how to carry out the CEE and which energy to deliver.

The vast majority of defibrillators currently on the market are models that deliver a shock with a biphasic wave.

The recommended energy with these devices is generally between 150 and 200 Joules. In the case of a need for repeated electric shocks, the energy is either constant or increasing according to the settings [11].

In the case of a manual biphasic defibrillator, it is recommended that the 1st shock be delivered with a minimum energy of 150 J, and then if necessary, subsequent shocks can be delivered with increasing energy up to 360 J [11]. (Appendix 3)

6.2   Conduct after EWC :

Each electric shock should be followed by immediate resumption of external cardiac massage, with total interruption of chest compressions not to exceed 5 seconds to keep interruption of cardiac massage to a minimum [11].

A percentage of 66% of the trained population assured that CPR should be resumed immediately after delivering the shock versus only 38% in the untrained group.

7.   Etiologies of CA:

The etiologies of CA are multiple and can be divided into 2 entities:

- Cardiac causes, which in adults account for about 80% of strokes: acute coronary syndrome, valvular disease, cardiomyopathy, congenital heart disease or rhythm disorder [11].

- Extracardial causes which are generally represented by neurological, traumatic, toxic or respiratory hypoxic etiologies: pulmonary embolism, diabetic decompensation, epilepsy, ... [11].

8.   Reversible causes *:*

Etiologies are classically memorable in "4H and 4T", must be known because they are reversible and require relatively simple treatments, in per and/or post-RCP:

- Hypoxia, Hypovolemia, Hypo/hyperkalemia, Hypothermia

- Thrombosis (coronary or pulmonary), suffocating pneumoThorax, Tamponnade and inToxications [11].

In our study, a majority ranging from 62% to 78% of trained respondents correctly cited the 4Hs and 4Ts, while the percentage for the same response ranged from 24% to 48% for untrained respondents.

Recognizing reversible causes of CA is very important to treat them immediately to improve the vital prognosis, simulation with scenarios including ACBO with reversible cause explains the superior knowledge of trained personnel.

9.   Etiologies of CA according to chronology:

Depending on the chronology, the causes of a CA are different:

<u>At the beginning of anaesthesia</u>: the CA must first evoke a warning sign related to an intubation

error (oesophageal intubation) or to a malposition of the probe or any other cause previously described, but also a vagal reflex or a ventricular rhythm disorder. After induction, from the first minutes of artificial ventilation, in the presence of a precarious hemodynamic state (hypovolemia, vasodilatation), CA may be due to the negative inotropic effect of anesthetic drugs, to rebreathing collapse, to an error in the administration of inhaled gases or in the intravenous dosage of the narcotic, or finally to a suffocating pneumothorax under machine. More rarely, it may be an anaphylactic or anaphylactoid reaction, especially observed with curares (depolarizing: Succinylcholine or non depolarizing: Atracurium or others). The latter type of agents may give rise to histaminoliberation reactions resulting in AC after bradycardia associated with bronchospasm.

10.   Cardiac arrest during laparoscopy:

CA during pneumoperitoneum should raise the possibility of massive gas embolism (GE). The best diagnostic tool is carbon dioxide end-tidal pressure (PETCO2) monitoring. If PETCO2 increases moderately after the creation of a carbon dioxide (CO2) pneumoperitoneum, its abrupt decrease or even collapse reflects massive GE.

Auscultation of both lung fields with a stethoscope detects a rough sound in case of significant EG. Transesophageal ultrasound reveals the passage of gas into the right atrium and detects small volume gas emboli [12].

Such a diagnosis justifies the immediate cessation of insufflation and exsufflation, the administration of nitrous oxide (N2O) must be stopped, ventilation is done with pure oxygen with an increase in the tidal volume and the introduction of positive pressure. The patient is placed in the Trendelenburg position with left lateralization. If a central line is in place, it is legitimate to attempt to aspirate a fraction of the embolus. Macromolecular volume expansion should be offered. CPR itself has no particularity except that the objective of MCE in this indication is to fractionate the emboli [12].

In our study, a rate of 70% of the simulation-trained population cited gas embolism as a cause of CA during laparoscopy versus 54% of the untrained population.

Simulation training allows the participants to be confronted with various examples of surgical procedures that can be complicated by BCAs with certain specificities of management and treatment such as gas embolism, fat embolism, cement embolism, amniotic embolism and even cardiac arrest following massive hemorrhage or in a patient in prone position, which will reinforce the skills of ASDs and MARs in dealing with BCAs in these various contexts.

11. Specific care for the post-CA period:

The primary goal of care in the post-CAE period is to achieve survival with little or no neurological sequelae, maintain homeostasis, especially metabolically, and methods to optimize oxygen delivery and treat hemodynamic consequences.

The gasometric objectives include obtaining an arterial saturation (SPO2) > 92% and normocapnia. Arterial hypotension is deleterious. The optimal blood pressure (BP) level in this situation must be adapted to the patient's terrain and previous blood pressure.

Therapeutic hypothermia can also be proposed but should be discussed on a case-by-case basis, taking into account the individual risk-benefit ratio, in which case it is necessary to use curarization in combination with sedation. (Sedation has not been shown to have a neuroprotective effect and should not be used routinely unless it is necessary for the use of therapeutic hypothermia).

Clinical work to evaluate the value of brain monitoring procedures should be encouraged in the context of post cardiac arrest syndrome [9].

In this context, a very small percentage of non-simulation trained personnel (10% and 2%) mentioned the stability of hemodynamic status and brain function as important elements of this management. Indeed, theoretical training alone is insufficient to ensure adequate management of an ACBO from its onset to the post-recovery period.

12. Importance of simulation training in the management of OGCA :

Simulation training has a crucial role in the management of critical situations in the operating room, it is one of the main ways to maintain and improve the quality of work of health workers [13].

In particular, it allows for better management of cardiac arrest in the operating room via various scenarios that confront the learner (TSA and MAR) with different situations that may be encountered in reality.

Simulation in the medical field is a learning method. The motivations for simulation are first of all ethical: "Never the first time on the patient! Simulation is also beneficial in learning communication skills and acquiring theoretical knowledge. It is an essential means of maintaining patient safety by limiting the risk of errors. It concerns the learning of technical gestures with the most realistic models possible [14].

CONCLUSION

CONCLUSION

Cardiac arrest remains a major public health problem and its occurrence in the operating room is a serious complication of anesthesia.

Simulation training allows the updating of knowledge and the maintenance of skills, but also the learning of how to deal with possible crisis situations in the operating room, particularly ACBO.

The aim of this work was to evaluate the theoretical and practical knowledge of medical and paramedical staff in anaesthesia and resuscitation in the management of a patient suffering from cardiac arrest in the operating theatre and to highlight the value of training by simulation.

This was a descriptive and analytical study comparing two groups of ASDs and MARs, 50 of whom had simulation training in CBOT and 50 of whom did not have simulation training.

The results of our study showed that the personnel trained by simulation have a superior knowledge concerning the diagnosis of ACBO, the particularities of the checklist and its different items, the modalities of performing chest compressions, ventilation and defibrillation in case of ACBO but also the pharmacological treatment to be administered.

The different causes of cardiac arrest, particularly the reversible causes and the steps to take after recovery from cardiac arrest, were also better known by the personnel trained by simulation.

In conclusion, simulation training is an important tool that can improve the knowledge of ASD and MAR in crisis situations in the operating room and particularly in the case of ACBO and thus reduce the morbidity and mortality of this pathology.

The inclusion of simulation in the continuing education of medical and paramedical anaesthesia staff is therefore necessary.

BIBLIOGRAPHY

Bibliographic references

[1]: Gueugniaud PY, Bertrand C, Savary D, Hubert H. Cardiac arrest in France: why a national register? Presse Med 2011

[2]: WHO (World Health Organization): Safer surgery saves lives

[3] : SFAR (French Society of Anaesthesia and Intensive Care): Recommendation for the organization of the management of vital emergencies in hospitals.

[4] : SFAR : COGNITIVE AIDS IN ANESTHESIA

[5] ANNE-LAURE CONSTANT: CARDIOPULMONARY ARREST IN THE OPERATING ROOM: IDENTIFICATION OF DETERMINANTS OF FUNCTIONAL PROGNOSIS AT 3 MONTHS. HUMAN MEDICINE AND PATHOLOGY. 2014.

[6]: Idris AH, Guffey D, Pepe PE; Resuscitation Outcomes Consortium Investigators. Chest compression rates and survival following out-of-hospital cardiac arrest

[7]: Eftestol T, Sunde K, Steen PA. Effects of interrupting precordial compressions on the calculated probability of defibrillation success during out-of-hospital cardiac arrest. Circulation 2002

[8] : Pell JP, Sirel JM, Marsden AK: Presentation, management, and outcome of out of hospital cardiopulmonary arrest: comparison by underlying aetiology

[9]: FORMALIZED RECOMMENDATIONS OF EXPERTS Management of cardiac arrest SFAR (Société française d'anesthésie et de réanimation) and the SRLF (Société de réanimation de langue française)

[10]: ERC (European Resuscitation Council) Guidelines for Resuscitation: 2018 Update - Antiarrhythmic drugs for cardiac arrest

[12] : Conférences d'actualisation 1999, p. 25-42. 1999 Elsevier, Paris, and SFAR : Intraoperative circulatory arrest

[13]: WHO: CONTINUING TRAINING FOR HEALTH CARE PERSONNEL - A MANUAL FOR WORKSHOPS (Geneva 1990)

[14] : INTERET DE LA SIMULATION EN PEDIATRIE/ VALUE OF SIMULATION IN PEDIATRIC PANELD.ORIOT A.BOUREAU-VOULTOURY A.GHAZALI C.BREQUE M.SCEPI
D.ORIOT

ANNEXES

ANNEX 1

<table>
<tr><td colspan="2">ARRET CARDIAQUE EN SERVICE DE RÉANIMATION ADULTE</td></tr>
<tr>
<td>
☐ Appeler renfort médical - Tél: ....
☐ Noter l'heure   ....h........
☐ Désigner un leader
☐ Personne dédiée au chronomètre / rapport écrit
</td>
<td>
VERIFIER
☐ Validité de l'ACR (Scope, SPO2, EtCO2, pression)
☐ Absence de LATA
☐ Chariot d'urgence sur place / Plan dur
☐ Arrêt médicaments hypotenseurs
</td>
</tr>
</table>

<table>
<tr><td colspan="2">Réanimation IMMEDIATE et CONTINUE</td></tr>
<tr>
<td>
☐ MCE 100 / minute
☐ Dépression sternale ≥ 5 cm
☐ Décollement des mains du sternum entre les compressions
☐ Relai toutes les 2 min
</td>
<td>
ET
☐ VENTILATION sur Sonde ou Masque Facial / BAVU
☐ Mettre en FiO_2 1
☐ FR basse 10/min
☐ Patient intubé : vérifier Intubation, sinon : Intuber

☐ Vérification / Pose voie veineuse ou intra osseuse

☐ Monitorage (Scope, Pression invasive, $EtCO_2$)
</td>
</tr>
</table>

ASYSTOLIE	FV ou TV

☐ Adrénaline 1 mg IVD / 3 à 5 min	☐ CEE Biphasique 200. Monophasique 360J ☐ suivi de 2 min de RCP	**ACR REFRACTAIRE** ☐ Echec RCP: évaluer rapidement indication / faisabilité d'**assistance circulatoire extracorporelle**. Tel: ....
	Répéter **3 fois** si nécessaire	**REPRISE RYTHME SPONTANE** Discuter :
Evaluation / 2 min de l'efficacité de la RCP : ☐ $EtCO_2$ > 12 mm Hg ☐ PAD > 20 mm Hg ☐ reprise activité cardiaque efficace	**Après 3ème CEE** ☐ Adrénaline 1 mg IVD ☐ Amiodarone IVD 1ère dose = 300 mg 2ème dose = 150 mg (CI si intox A. Locaux)	☐ L'indication d'hypothermie thérapeutique (32 – 35°C) pendant 12 à 24h ☐ La nécessité d'une coronarographie ☐ La sédation post arrêt cardiaque (n'a pas démontré d'effet neuroprotecteur)

ANNEX 2

ACR SUR ASYSTOLIE AU BLOC OPÉRATOIRE

CONFIRMER

- ☐ Tracé plat: ——————
- ☐ Absence de pouls
- ☐ Effondrement capnie
- ☐ Noter l'heure: .... H ....min
- ☐ Designer le leader

INITIER

- ☐ RCP
  - 100- 120 Compressions /min
  - 5 - 6 cm de profondeur
  - Relaxation complète
  - Rotation: toutes les 3 minutes

Appel à l'aide
STOP Chirurgie

TRAITER

- ☐ Evaluer l'efficacité de la RCP
  - EtCO$_2$ (20 mmHg)
  - Pression artérielle sanglante diastolique > 20-40 mmHg

- ☐ Défibrillateur mis en place : pas de choc
- ☐ Adrénaline 1 mg / 3-5min
- ☐ Massage cardiaque externe en continu
- ☐ Intuber si non réalisé préalablement

VÉRIFIER

- ☐ FiO2 = 1, haut débit de gaz frais
- ☐ Ventilation protectrice FR 10/min
- ☐ Accès veineux disponible

RECHERCHER CAUSES
- ☐ Respiratoires
- ☐ Cardiovasculaires
- ☐ Métaboliques
- ☐ Anesthésiques
- ☐ Neurologiques

En cas d'arrêt cardiaque réfractaire:
Réanimation prolongée
Envisager une assistance cardio-circulatoire (ECLS/ECMO)

Références:
ERC Guidelines 2015. http://www.cprguidelines.eu/
Cardiac Arrest in the Operating Room. Janusz A.
http://www.esahq.org/~/media/ESA/Files/Refresher%20Courses/2012/Cardiac%20arrest%20in%20the%20operating%20room%20(2012).ashx
Arrêt cardio-circulatoire au bloc opératoire. Lena-Quintard D. Le Praticien en anesthesie réanimation.2015;19:136-42.
Recommandations formalisées d'experts. Prise en charge de l'arrêt cardiaque. AFAR.2007;26:1008-1019.

Réalisée en 2016 par le CAMR

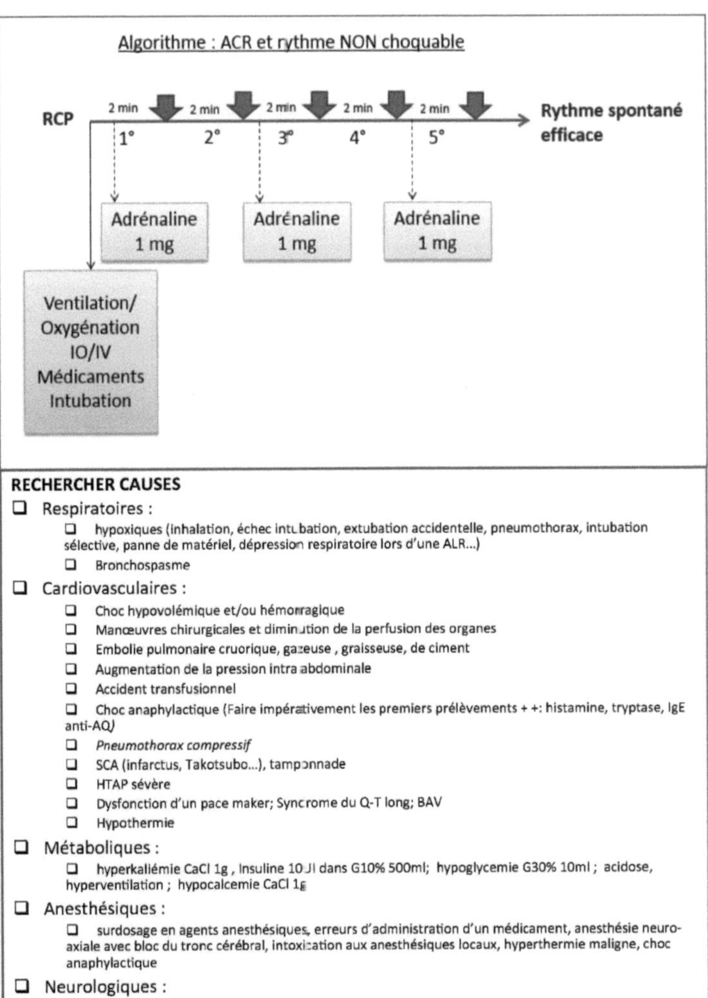

RECHERCHER CAUSES

❑ Respiratoires :
   ❑ hypoxiques (inhalation, échec intubation, extubation accidentelle, pneumothorax, intubation sélective, panne de matériel, dépression respiratoire lors d'une ALR...)
   ❑ Bronchospasme

❑ Cardiovasculaires :
   ❑ Choc hypovolémique et/ou hémorragique
   ❑ Manœuvres chirurgicales et diminution de la perfusion des organes
   ❑ Embolie pulmonaire cruorique, gazeuse , graisseuse, de ciment
   ❑ Augmentation de la pression intra abdominale
   ❑ Accident transfusionnel
   ❑ Choc anaphylactique (Faire impérativement les premiers prélèvements + +: histamine, tryptase, IgE anti-AQ)
   ❑ *Pneumothorax compressif*
   ❑ SCA (infarctus, Takotsubo...), tamponnade
   ❑ HTAP sévère
   ❑ Dysfonction d'un pace maker; Syncrome du Q-T long; BAV
   ❑ Hypothermie

❑ Métaboliques :
   ❑ hyperkaliémie CaCl 1g , Insuline 10 UI dans G10% 500ml; hypoglycemie G30% 10ml ; acidose, hyperventilation ; hypocalcemie CaCl 1g

❑ Anesthésiques :
   ❑ surdosage en agents anesthésiques, erreurs d'administration d'un médicament, anesthésie neuro-axiale avec bloc du tronc cérébral, intoxication aux anesthésiques locaux, hyperthermie maligne, choc anaphylactique

❑ Neurologiques :
   ❑ accident vasculaire cérébral, hypertension intra crânienne

APPENDIX 3

ACR SUR TV OU FV AU BLOC OPÉRATOIRE

CONFIRMER

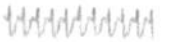

- [ ] ᜉᜉᜉᜉᜉᜉ ou ᜉᜉᜉᜉᜉᜉ
- [ ] Absence de pouls
- [ ] Effondrement capnie
- [ ] Noter l'heure: ……… H ………min
- [ ] Designer le leader

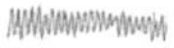

INITIER

- [ ] RCP
  - 100 - 120 Compressions /min
  - 5-6 cm de profondeur
  - Relaxation complète
  - Rotation: toutes les 3 minutes

Appel à l'aide
STOP Chirurgie

TRAITER

- [ ] Evaluer l'efficacité de la RCP
  - $EtCO_2$
  - Pression artérielle sanglante diastolique > 20-40 mmHg

- [ ] Défibrillateur 200 J biphasique : 1er Choc

  2ème Choc ⟩ RCP 2min

  3ème Choc ⟩ RCP 2min

  4ème Choc ⟩ RCP 2min
  Adrénaline 1mg + Cordarone 300mg IVD
- [ ] Renouveler Adrénaline 1mg/3min
- [ ] Renouveler Cordarone 150mg IVD + relais Cordarone 900mg/24h IVSE

VÉRIFIER

- [ ] FiO2 = 1, haut débit de gaz frais
- [ ] Ventilation protectrice FR 10/min
- [ ] Accès veineux disponible

RECHERCHER CAUSES

- [ ] Respiratoires
- [ ] Cardiovasculaires
- [ ] Métaboliques
- [ ] Anesthésiques
- [ ] Neurologiques

Références:
ERC Guidelines 2015. http://www.cprguidelines.eu/
Cardiac Arrest in the Operating Room. Janusz A.
http://www.esaho.org/~/media/ESA/Files/Refresher%20Courses/2012/Cardiac%20arrest%20in%20the%20operating%20room%20(2012).ashx
Arrêt cardio-circulatoire au bloc opératoire. Lena-Quintard D. Le Praticien en anesthesie réanimation.2015;19:136-42.
Recommandations formalisées d'experts. Prise en charge de l'arrêt cardiaque. AFAR.2007;26:1008-1019.

SFAR Société Française d'Anesthésie et de Réanimation

Réalisée en 2016 par le CAMR

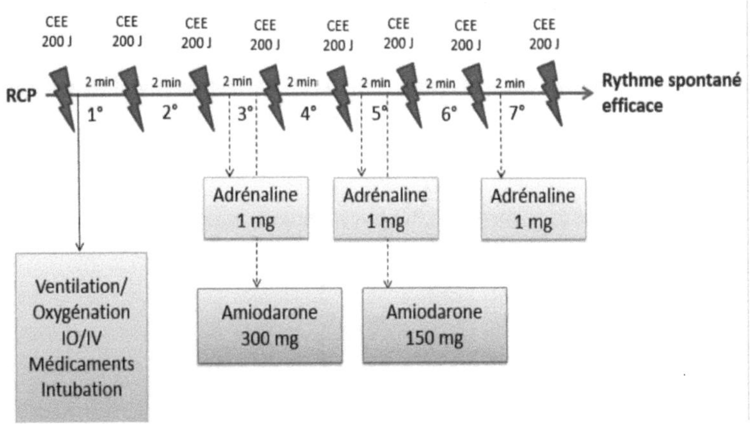

RECHERCHER CAUSES

☐ Respiratoires :

- ☐ hypoxiques (inhalation, échec intubation, extubation accidentelle, pneumothorax, intubation sélective, panne de matériel, dépression respiratoire lors d'une ALR…)
- ☐ Bronchospasme

☐ Cardiovasculaires :

- ☐ Choc hypovolémique et/ou hémorragique
- ☐ Manœuvres chirurgicales et diminution de la perfusion des organes
- ☐ Embolie pulmonaire cruorique, gazeuse , graisseuse, de ciment
- ☐ Augmentation de la pression intra abdominale
- ☐ Accident transfusionnel
- ☐ Choc anaphylactique (Faire impérativement les premiers prélèvements + + : histamine, tryptase, IgE anti-AQ)
- ☐ Pneumothorax compressif
- ☐ SCA (infarctus, Takotsubo…), tamponnade
- ☐ HTAP sévère
- ☐ Dysfonction d'un pace maker; Syndrome du Q-T long; BAV
- ☐ Hypothermie

☐ Métaboliques :

- ☐ hyperkaliémie CaCl 1g , Insuline 10UI dans G10% 500ml; hypoglycemie G30% 10ml ; acidose, hyperventilation ; hypocalcemie CaCl 1g

☐ Anesthésiques :

- ☐ surdosage en agents anesthésiques, erreurs d'administration d'un médicament, anesthésie neuro-axiale avec bloc du tronc cérébral, intoxication aux anesthésiques locaux, hyperthermie maligne, choc anaphylactique

☐ Neurologiques :

- ☐ accident vasculaire cérébral, hypertension intra crânienne

ANNEX 4

We are students in anesthesia and resuscitation at the Central University.

As part of our final year project, we are carrying out a survey of medical and paramedical staff in anaesthesia and intensive care, with the aim of highlighting their skills and knowledge of the protocol to be followed in the event of intraoperative cardiac arrest.

Please take a few minutes to complete this questionnaire, which will remain anonymous and confidential.

. Hospital: ....

. Sex :

☐ Female

☐ Male

. Function :

☐ Senior in Anesthesia and Resuscitation

☐ Resident in anesthesia and resuscitation

☐ Anesthesia and resuscitation technician

. Seniority in the function :

☐ < 5 years

☐ 5 to 10 years

☐ > 10 years

1) Have you ever had specific training in the management of cardiac arrest in the operating room?

☐ Yes ☐ No

2) In your opinion, are there any particulars in the operating room checklist that should be prepared on a daily basis to be always prepared in case of a cardiac arrest?

☐ Yes ☐ No

. If 'Yes' which ones?

....

....

3) What is the first warning sign of cardiac arrest in the operating room?

....

....

....

4) Have you ever had a cardiac arrest during surgery?

☐ Yes ☐ No

5) What is your response to this situation?

....

....

6) How many chest compressions should be performed during external CPR?

☐ 15

☐ 30

☐According to the victim's improvement

7) What do you think the compression/ventilation ratio is?

☐ 30/2

☐ 30/3

☐ 15/2

8) How to ventilate a patient in cardiac arrest:

☐ Vt: 6-7ml/kg, Inspiratory frequency: 10/min, Insp time: 2sec

☐ Vt: 4-5ml/kg, Inspiratory rate: 6/min, Insp time: 1sec

☐ Vt: 10-12ml/kg, Inspiratory frequency: 40/min, Insp time: 3sec

9) What is the proper depth of chest compressions in adults for cardiac massage to be effective?

☐ 6 to 10 cm

☐ 5 to 6 cm

☐ 10 to 15 cm

10) What is the frequency of compressions for cardiac massage?

☐ 50 to 60/min

☐ 100 to 120/min

☐ 75 to 80/min

11) What is the drug of choice for cardiac arrest?

☐ Adrenaline

☐ Noradrenaline

☐ Dobutamine

. Name the appropriate dose :

....

12) This drug is to be administered every :

☐ 4 cycles

☐ 2 cycles

☐ 6 cycles

13) What are some of the etiologies that can cause cardiac arrest during induction?

....

14) What can cause cardiac arrest during laparoscopy?

....

15) What type of defibrillator is available in your workplace?

☐ Automated external

☐ Semi-automatic

16) Define a shockable rhythm?

17) What to do immediately after delivering the shock?

....

18) When should an anti-arrhythmic be administered?

☐ Before the 3rd or 4th external electric shock

☐ After the 3rd or 4th external electric shock

19) What are the reversible causes of cardiac arrest?

....

....

...

20) If hypothermia is present, should CPR be withheld until the victim is rewarmed?

☐ Yes

☐ No

21) After the patient is stabilized, what is the specific care of the post-cardiac arrest period?

....

...

We thank you once again for your contribution

Summary

Introduction:

Cardiac arrest, also known as sudden adult death or cardiopulmonary arrest, is an abrupt cessation of heart muscle contractions and breathing by the patient, resulting in an interruption of perfusion to the body's vital organs. The occurrence of cardiac arrest in the operating room (ACBO) is a rare but very serious situation in anesthesia.

Deaths from cardiac arrest are most often due to a lack of prompt attention to the victim, mainly because of delayed diagnosis.

Objectives: To evaluate the knowledge of technicians and doctors in anaesthesia and resuscitation regarding the management of ACBO and to develop the interest of training by simulation in order to refresh the knowledge and develop the skills of the intervening parties.

Materials and methods:

This is a prospective, analytical and comparative study in the form of an anonymous multi-centre questionnaire. We distributed 100 questionnaires to anaesthesia staff (doctors and technicians): 50 for simulation-trained staff and 50 for non-simulation-trained staff.

Results:

Of the respondents who had received simulation training, 82% responded that the number of chest compressions was 30 versus 42% of the untrained group. This difference was statistically significant (p=0.01). Simulation-trained personnel also had better knowledge of the number of compressions and the depth of compressions (p=0.01).

The adequate dose of epinephrine was better known by those trained in simulation (90 vs 72%, p=0.04). A majority ranging from 62% to 78% of trained respondents correctly cited reversible causes of cardiac arrest, this percentage ranged from 24% to 48% for untrained respondents, this difference was not statistically significant. Thirty (30%) of the trained simulation respondents cited hemodynamic stability as the primary resuscitative measure after CA recovery followed by neuroprotection (14%) and maintenance of homeostasis (8%). The rate of untrained respondents who maintained hemodynamic stability and provided neuroprotection was lower.

Conclusion:

Simulation training is an important tool that can improve the knowledge of ASDs and MARs in crisis situations in the operating room and particularly in cases of CABG and thus reduce the morbidity and mortality of this pathology.

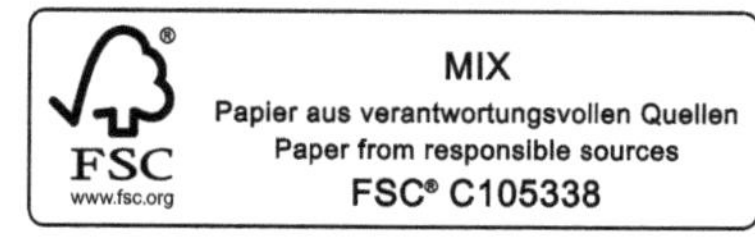

Printed by Books on Demand GmbH, Norderstedt / Germany